Pegan Diet Delights

Super Tasty, Affordable and Easy Recipes for
your Snack and Dessert Dishes

Kimberly Solis

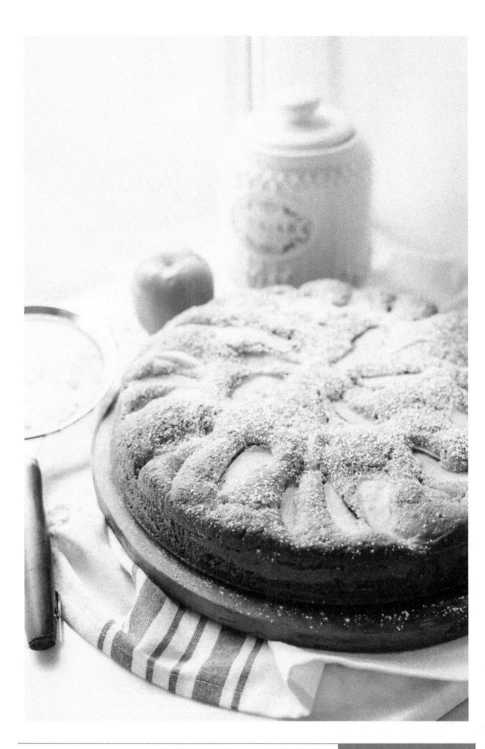

Table of Contents

Pear Croustade

Preparation Time: 30 Minutes

Cooking Time: 60 Minutes

Servings: 10

Ingredients:

- 1 cup plus 1 tbsp. all-purpose flour, divided
- 4 ½ tbsps. sugar, divided
- 1/8 tsp salt
- 6 tbsps. unsalted butter, chilled, cut into ½ inch cubes
- 1 large-sized egg, separated
- 1 1/2 tbsps. ice-cold water
- 3 firm, ripe pears (Bosc), peeled, cored, sliced into ¼ inch slices 1 tbsp. fresh lemon juice
- 1/3 tsp ground allspice
- 1 tsp anise seeds

Directions:

1. Pour 1 cup of flour, 1 ½ Tbsps. of sugar, butter, and salt into a food processor and combine the ingredients by pulsing.

2. Whisk the yolk of the egg and ice water in a separate bowl. Mix the egg mixture with the flour mixture. It will form a dough, wrap it, and set aside for an hour.

3. Set the oven to 400°F.

4. Mix the pear, sugar, leftover flour, allspice, anise seed, and lemon juice in a large bowl to make a filling.

5. Arrange the filling on the center of the dough.

6. Bake for about 40 minutes. Cool for about 15 minutes before serving.

Nutrition:

Calories: 498kcal

Carbs: 32g

Fat: 32g

Protein: 18g

Melomakarona

Preparation Time: 20 Minutes

Cooking Time: 45 Minutes

Servings: 20

Ingredients:

- 4 cups of sugar, divided
- 4 cups of water
- 1 cup plus 1 tbsp. honey, divided
- 1 (2-inch) strip orange peel, pith removed
- 1 cinnamon stick
- ½ cup extra-virgin olive oil
- ¼ cup unsalted butter,
- ¼ cup Metaxa brandy or any other brandy
- 1 tbsp. grated
- Orange zest
- ¾ cup of orange juice
- ¼ tsp baking soda
- 3 cups pastry flour
- ¾ cup fine semolina flour

- 1 ½ tsp baking powder

- 4 tsp ground cinnamon, divided

- 1 tsp ground cloves, divided

- 1 cup finely chopped walnut

- 1/3 cup brown sugar

Directions:

1. Mix 3 ½ cups of sugar, 1 cup honey, orange peel, cinnamon stick, and water in a pot and heat it for about 10 minutes.

2. Mix the sugar, oil, and butter for about minutes, then add the brandy, leftover honey, and zest. Then add a mixture of baking soda and orange juice. Mix thoroughly.

3. In a distinct bowl, blend the pastry flour, baking powder, semolina, 2 tsp of cinnamon, and ½ tsp. of cloves. Add the mixture to the mixer slowly. Run the mixer until the ingredients form a dough. Cover and set aside for 30 minutes.

4. Set the oven to 350°F

5. With your palms, form small oval balls from the dough. Make a total of forty balls.

6. Bake the cookie balls for 30 minutes, then drop them in the prepared syrup.

7. Create a mixture with the walnuts, leftover cinnamon, and cloves. Spread the mixture on the top of the baked cookies.

8. Serve the cookies or store them in a closed-lid container.

Nutrition:

Calories: 294kcal

Carbs: 44g

Fat: 12g

Protein: 3g

Fried Honey Balls

Preparation Time: 20 Minutes

Cooking Time: 45 Minutes

Servings: 10

Ingredients:

- 2 cups of sugar
- 1 cup of water
- 1 cup honey
- 1 ½ cups tepid water
- 1 tbsp. brown sugar
- ¼ cup of vegetable oil
- 1 tbsp. active dry yeast
- 1 ½ cups all-purpose flour, 1 cup cornstarch, ½ tsp salt
- Vegetable oil for frying
- 1 ½ cups chopped walnuts
- ¼ cup ground cinnamon

Directions:

1. Boil the sugar and water on medium heat. Add honey after 10 minutes. cool and set aside.

2. Mix the tepid water, oil, brown sugar,' and yeast in a large bowl. Allow it to sit for 10 minutes. In a distinct bowl, blend the flour, salt, and cornstarch. With your hands mix the yeast and the flour to make a wet dough. Cover and set aside for 2 hours.

3. Fry in oil at 350°F. Use your palm to measure the sizes of the dough as they are dropped in the frying pan. Fry each batch for about 3-4 minutes.

4. Immediately the loukoumades are done frying, drop them in the prepared syrup.

5. Serve with cinnamon and walnuts.

Nutrition:

Calories: 355kcal

Carbs: 64g

Fat: 7g

Protein: 6g

Crème Caramel

Preparation Time: 60 Minutes

Cooking Time: 60 Minutes

Servings: 12

Ingredients:

- 5 cups of whole milk
- 2 tsp vanilla extract
- 8 large egg yolks
- 4 large-sized eggs
- 2 cups sugar, divided
- ¼ cup of water

Directions:

1. Preheat the oven to 350°F

2. Heat the milk with medium heat wait for it to be scalded.

3. Mix 1 cup of sugar and eggs in a bowl and add it to the eggs.

4. With a nonstick pan on high heat, boil the water and remaining sugar. Do not stir, instead whirl the pan. When the sugar forms caramel, divide it into ramekins.

5. Divide the egg mixture into the ramekins and place in a baking pan. Increase water to the pan until it is half full. Bake for 30 minutes.

6. Remove the ramekins from the baking pan, cool, then refrigerate for at least 8 hours.

7. Serve.

Nutrition:

Calories: 110kcal

Carbs: 21g

Fat: 1g

Protein: 2g

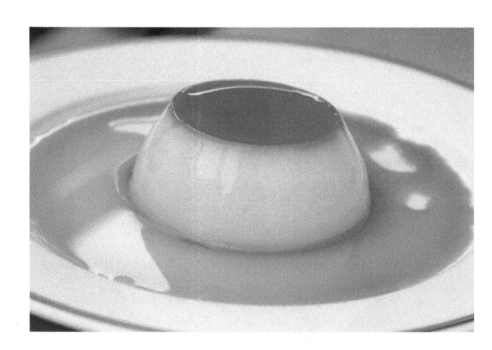

Galaktoboureko

Preparation Time: 30 Minutes

Cooking Time: 90 Minutes

Servings: 12

Ingredients:

- 4 cups sugar, divided
- 1 tbsp. fresh lemon juice
- 1 cup of water
- 1 Tbsp. plus 1 ½ tsp grated lemon zest, divided into 10 cups
- Room temperature whole milk
- 1 cup plus 2 tbsps. unsalted butter, melted and divided into 2
- Tbsps. vanilla extract
- 7 large-sized eggs
- 1 cup of fine semolina
- 1 package phyllo, thawed and at room temperature

Directions:

1. Preheat oven to 350°F
2. Mix 2 cups of sugar, lemon juice, 1 ½ tsp of lemon zest, and water. Boil over medium heat. Set aside.

3. Mix the milk, 2 Tbsps. of butter, and vanilla in a pot and put-on medium heat. Remove from heat when milk is scalded

4. Mix the eggs and semolina in a bowl, then add the mixture to the scalded milk. Put the egg-milk mixture on medium heat. Stir until it forms a custard-like material.

5. Brush butter on each sheet then arrange all over the baking pan until everywhere is covered. Spread the custard on the bottom pile phyllo

6. Arrange the buttered phyllo all over the top of the custard until every inch is covered.

7. Bake for about 40 minutes. cover the top of the pie with all the prepared syrup. Serve.

Nutrition:

Calories: 393kcal

Carbs: 55g

Fat: 15g

Protein: 8g

Kourabiedes Almond Cookies

Preparation Time: 20 Minutes

Cooking Time: 50 Minutes

Servings: 20

Ingredients:

- 1 ½ cups unsalted butter, clarified, at room temperature 2 cups

- Confectioners' sugar, divided

- 1 large egg yolk

- 2 tbsps. brandy

- 1 1/2 tsp baking powder

- 1 tsp vanilla extract

- 5 cups all-purpose flour, sifted

- 1 cup roasted almonds, chopped

Directions:

1. Preheat the oven to 350°F

2. Thoroughly mix butter and ½ cup of sugar in a bowl. Add in the egg after a while. Create a brandy mixture by mixing the brandy and baking powder. Add the mixture to the egg, add vanilla, then keep beating until the ingredients are properly blended

3. Add flour and almonds to make a dough.

4. Roll the dough to form crescent shapes. You should be able to get about 40 pieces. Place the pieces on a baking sheet, then bake in the oven for 25 minutes.

5. Allow the cookies to cool, then coat them with the remaining confectioner's sugar.

6. Serve.

Nutrition:

Calories: 102kcal

Carbs: 10g

Fat: 7g

Protein: 2g

Ekmek Kataifi

Preparation Time: 30 Minutes

Cooking Time: 45 Minutes

Servings: 10

Ingredients:

- 1 cup of sugar
- 1 cup of water
- 2 (2-inch) strips lemon peel, pith removed
- 1 tbsp. fresh lemon juice
- ½ cup plus 1 tbsp. unsalted butter, melted
- ½lbs. frozen kataifi pastry, thawed, at room temperature
- 2 ½ cups whole milk
- ½ tsp. ground mastiha
- 2 large eggs
- ¼ cup fine semolina
- 1 tsp. of cornstarch
- ¼ cup of sugar
- ½ cup sweetened coconut flakes
- 1 cup whipping cream

- 1 tsp. vanilla extract

- 1 tsp. powdered milk

- 3 tbsps. of confectioners' sugar

- ½ cup chopped unsalted pistachios

Directions:

1. Set the oven to 350°F. Grease the baking pan with 1. Tbsp of butter.

2. Put a pot on medium heat, then add water, sugar, lemon juice, lemon peel. Leave to boil for about 10 minutes. Reserve.

3. Untangle the kataifi, coat with the leftover butter, then place in the baking pan.

4. Mix the milk and mastiha, then place it on medium heat. Remove from heat when the milk is scalded, then cool the mixture.

5. Mix the eggs, cornstarch, semolina, and sugar in a bowl, stir thoroughly, then whisk the cooled milk mixture into the bowl.

6. Transfer the egg and milk mixture to a pot and place on heat. Wait for it to thicken like custard, then add the coconut flakes and cover it with a plastic wrap. Cool.

7. Spread the cooled custard-like material over the kataifi. Place in the refrigerator for at least 8 hours.

8. Strategically remove the kataifi from the pan with a knife. Take it away in such a way that the mold faces up.

9. Whip a cup of cream, add 1 tsp. vanilla, 1tsp. powdered milk, and 3 tbsps. Of sugar. Spread the mixture all over the custard, wait for it to harden, then flip and add the leftover cream mixture to the kataifi side.

10. Serve.

Nutrition:

Calories: 649kcal

Carbs: 37g

Fat: 52g

Protein: 11g

Revani Syrup Cake

Preparation Time: 30 Minutes

Cooking Time: 3 Hours

Servings: 24

Ingredients:

- 1 tbsp. unsalted butter

- 2 tbsps. all-purpose flour

- 1 cup ground rusk or bread crumbs

- 1 cup fine semolina flour

- ¾ cup ground toasted almonds

- 3 tsp baking powder

- 16 large eggs

- 2 tbsps. vanilla extract

- 3 cups of sugar, divided

- 3 cups of water

- 5 (2-inch) strips lemon peel, pith removed

- 3 tbsps. fresh lemon juice

- 1 oz of brandy

Directions:

1. Preheat the oven to 350°F. Grease the baking pan with 1 Tbsp. of butter and flour.

2. Mix the rusk, almonds, semolina, baking powder in a bowl.

3. In another bowl, mix the eggs, 1 cup of sugar, vanilla, and whisk with an electric mixer for about 5 minutes. Add the semolina mixture to the eggs and stir.

4. Pour the stirred batter into the greased baking pan and place in the preheated oven.

5. With the remaining sugar, lemon peels, and water make the syrup by boiling the mixture on medium heat. Add the lemon juice after 6 minutes, then cook for 3 minutes. Remove the lemon peels and set the syrup aside.

6. After the cake is done in the oven, spread the syrup over the cake.

7. Cut the cake as you please and serve.

Nutrition:

Calories: 348kcal

Carbs: 55g

Fat: 9g

Protein: 5g

Almonds and Oats Pudding

Preparation Time: 10 Minutes

Cooking Time: 15 Minutes

Servings: 4

Ingredients:

- 1 tablespoon lemon juice

- Zest of 1 lime

- 1 and ½ cups of almond milk

- 1 teaspoon almond extract

- ½ cup oats

- 2 tablespoons stevia

- ½ cup silver almonds, chopped

Directions:

1. In a pan, blend the almond milk plus the lime zest and the other ingredients, whisk, bring to a simmer and cook over medium heat for 15 minutes.

2. Split the mix into bowls then serve cold.

Nutrition:

Calories 174

Fat 12.1

Fiber 3.2

Carbs 3.9

Protein 4.8

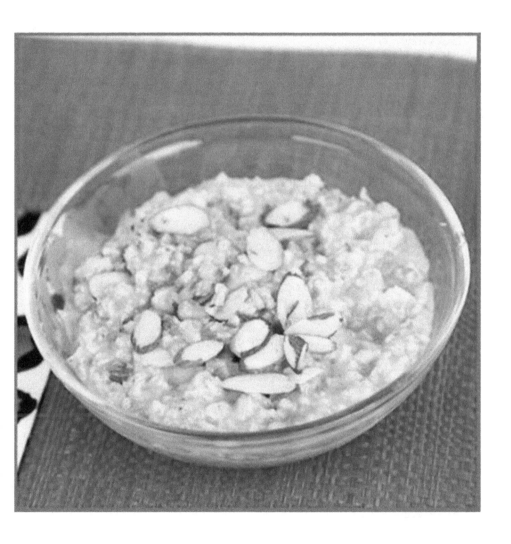

Chocolate Cups

Preparation Time: 2 Hours

Cooking Time: 0 Minutes

Servings: 6

Ingredients:

- ½ cup avocado oil

- 1 cup, chocolate, melted

- 1 teaspoon matcha powder

- 3 tablespoons stevia

Directions:

1. In a bowl, mix the chocolate with the oil and the rest of the ingredients.

2. Whisk well and divide into cups.

3. Keep in the freezer for 2 hours before serving.

Nutrition:

Calories 174

Fat 9.1

Fiber 2.2

Carbs 3.9

Protein 2.8

Mango Bowls

Preparation Time: 30 Minutes

Cooking Time: 0 Minutes

Servings: 4

Ingredients:

- 3 cups mango, cut into medium chunks
- ½ cup of coconut water
- ¼ cup stevia
- 1 teaspoon vanilla extract

Directions:

1. In a blender, blend the mango plus the rest of the ingredients, pulse well.
2. Divide into bowls and serve cold.

Nutrition:

Calories 122

Fat 4

Fiber 5.3

Carbs 6.6

Protein 4.5

Cocoa and Pears Cream

Preparation Time: 10 Minutes

Cooking Time: 0 Minutes

Servings: 4

Ingredients:

- 2 cups heavy creamy
- 1/3 cup stevia
- ¾ cup cocoa powder
- 6 ounces dark chocolate, chopped
- Zest of 1 lemon
- 2 pears, chopped

Directions:

1. In a blender, blend the cream plus the stevia and the rest of the ingredients.
2. Blend well.
3. Divide into cups and serve cold.

Nutrition:
Calories 172
Fat 5.6
Fiber 3.5
Carbs 7.6
Protein 4

Pineapple Pudding

Preparation Time: 10 Minutes

Cooking Time: 40 Minutes

Servings: 4

Ingredients:

- 3 cups almond flour
- ¼ cup olive oil
- 1 teaspoon vanilla extract
- 2 and ¼ cups stevia
- 3 eggs, whisked
- 1 and ¼ cup natural apple sauce
- 2 teaspoons baking powder
- 1 and ¼ cups of almond milk
- 2 cups pineapple, chopped
- Cooking spray

Directions:

1. In a bowl, blend the almond flour plus the oil and the rest of the ingredients except the cooking spray and stir well.

2. Grease a cake pan with the cooking spray, pour the pudding mix inside, introduce in the oven and bake at 370 degrees F for 40 minutes.

3. Serve the pudding cold.

Nutrition:

Calories 223

Fat 8.1

Fiber 3.4

Carbs 7.6

Protein 3.4

Lime Vanilla Fudge

Preparation Time: 3 Hours

Cooking Time: 0 Minutes

Servings: 6

Ingredients:

- 1/3 cup cashew butter
- 5 tablespoons lime juice
- ½ teaspoon lime zest, grated
- 1 tablespoons stevia

Directions:

1. In a bowl, mix the cashew butter with the other ingredients and whisk well.

2. Line a muffin tray with parchment paper, scoop 1 tablespoon of lime fudge mix in each of the muffin tins and keep in the freezer for 3 hours before serving.

Nutrition:

Calories 200

Fat 4.5

Fiber 3.4

Carbs 13.5

Protein 5

Mixed Berries Stew

Preparation Time: 10 Minutes

Cooking Time: 15 Minutes

Servings: 6

Ingredients:

- Zest of 1 lemon, grated
- Juice of 1 lemon
- ½ pint blueberries
- 1-pint strawberries halved
- 2 cups of water
- 2 tablespoons stevia

Directions:

1. In a pan, blend the berries plus the water, stevia and the other ingredients.
2. Bring to a simmer, cook over medium heat for 15 minutes.
3. Divide into bowls and serve cold.

Nutrition:

Calories 172

Fat 7

Fiber 3.4

Carbs 8

Protein 2.3

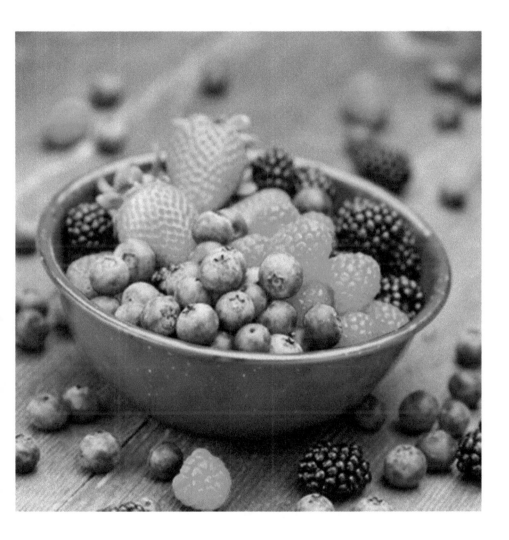

Orange and Apricots Cake

Preparation Time: 10 Minutes

Cooking Time: 20 Minutes

Servings: 8

Ingredients:

- ¾ cup stevia
- 2 cups almond flour
- ¼ cup olive oil
- ½ cup almond milk
- 1 teaspoon baking powder
- 2 eggs
- ½ teaspoon vanilla extract
- Juice and zest of 2 oranges
- 2 cups apricots, chopped

Directions:

1. In a bowl, blend the stevia plus the flour and the rest of the ingredients, whisk and pour into a cake pan lined with parchment paper.

2. Introduce in the oven at 375 degrees F, bake for 20 minutes.

3. Cool down, slice and serve.

Nutrition:

Calories 221

Fat 8.3

Fiber 3.4

Carbs 14.5

Protein 5

Blueberry Cake

Preparation Time: 10 Minutes

Cooking Time: 30 Minutes

Servings: 6

Ingredients:

- 2 cups almond flour
- 3 cups blueberries
- 1 cup walnuts, chopped
- 3 tablespoons stevia
- 1 teaspoon vanilla extract
- 2 eggs, whisked
- 2 tablespoons avocado oil
- 1 teaspoon baking powder
- Cooking spray

Directions:

1. In a bowl, blend the flour plus the blueberries, walnuts and the other ingredients except for the cooking spray, and stir well.

2. Grease a cake pan with the cooking spray, pour the cake mix inside, introduce everything in the oven at 350 degrees F and bake for 30 minutes.

3. Cool the cake down, slice and serve.

Nutrition:

Calories 225

Fat 9

Fiber 4.5

Carbs 10.2

Protein 4.5

Almond Peaches Mix

Preparation Time: 10 Minutes

Cooking Time: 10 Minutes

Servings: 4

Ingredients:

- 1/3 cup almonds, toasted
- 1/3 cup pistachios, toasted
- 1 teaspoon mint, chopped
- ½ cup of coconut water
- 1 teaspoon lemon zest, grated
- 4 peaches, halved
- 2 tablespoons stevia

Directions:

1. In a pan, combine the peaches with the stevia and the rest of the ingredients.
2. Simmer over medium heat for 10 minutes.
3. Divide into bowls and serve cold.

Nutrition:

Calories 135

Fat 4.1

Fiber 3.8

Carbs 4.1

Protein 2.3

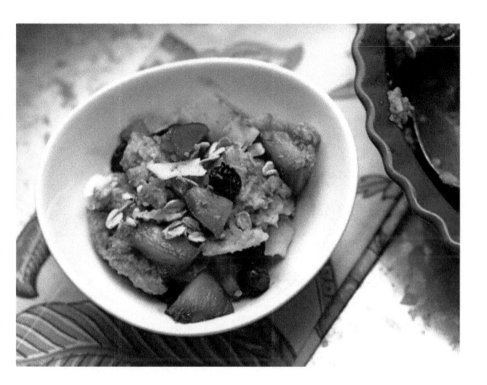

Spiced Peaches

Preparation Time: 5 minutes

Cooking Time: 10 minutes

Servings: 2

Ingredients:

- Canned peaches with juices – 1 cup

- Cornstarch – ½ tsp.

- Ground cloves – 1 tsp.

- Ground cinnamon – 1 tsp.

- Ground nutmeg – 1 tsp.

- Zest of ½ lemon

- Water – ½ cup

Directions:

1. Drain peaches.

2. Combine cinnamon, cornstarch, nutmeg, ground cloves, and lemon zest in a pan on the stove.

3. Heat on medium heat and add peaches.

4. Bring to a boil, decrease the heat then simmer for 10 minutes.

5. Serve.

Nutrition:

Calories: 70;

Fat: 0g;

Carb: 14g;

Phosphorus: 23mg;

Potassium: 176mg;

Sodium: 3mg;

Protein: 1g

Pumpkin Cheesecake Bar

Preparation Time: 10 minutes

Cooking Time: 50 minutes

Servings: 4

Ingredients:

- Unsalted butter – 2 ½ Tbsps.

- Cream cheese – 4 oz.

- All-purpose white flour – ½ cup

- Golden brown sugar – 3 Tbsps.

- Granulated sugar – ¼ cup

- Pureed pumpkin – ½ cup

- Egg whites - 2

- Ground cinnamon – 1 tsp.

- Ground nutmeg – 1 tsp.

- Vanilla extract – 1 tsp.

Directions:

1. Preheat the oven to 350F.

2. Mix brown sugar and flour in a container.

3. Mix in the butter to form 'breadcrumbs.'

4. Place ¾ of this mixture in a dish.

5. Bake in the oven for 15 minutes. Remove and cool.

6. Lightly whisk the egg and fold in the cream cheese, sugar, pumpkin, cinnamon, nutmeg, and vanilla until smooth.

7. Pour this mixture over the oven-baked base and sprinkle with the rest of the breadcrumbs from earlier.

8. Bake for 30 to 35 minutes more.

9. Cool, slice, and serve.

Nutrition:

Calories: 248;

Fat: 13g;

Carb: 33g;

Phosphorus: 67mg;

Potassium: 96mg;

Sodium: 146mg;

Protein: 4g

Blueberry Mini Muffins

Preparation Time: 10 minutes

Cooking Time: 35 minutes

Servings: 4

Ingredients:

- Egg whites – 3

- All-purpose white flour – ¼ cup

- Coconut flour – 1 Tbsp.

- Baking soda – 1 tsp.

- Nutmeg – 1 Tbsp. grated

- Vanilla extract – 1 tsp.

- Stevia – 1 tsp.

- Fresh blueberries – ¼ cup

Directions:

1. Preheat the oven to 325F.

2. Mix all the ingredients in a bowl.

3. Divide the batter into four and spoon into a lightly oiled muffin tin.

4. Bake in the oven for 15 to 20 minutes or until cooked through.

5. Cool and serve.

Nutrition:

Calories: 62;

Fat: 0g;

Carb: 9g;

Phosphorus: 103mg;

Potassium: 65mg;

Sodium: 62mg;

Protein: 4g;

Vanilla Custard

Preparation Time: 7 minutes

Cooking Time: 10 minutes

Servings: 10

Ingredients:

- Egg – 1
- Vanilla – 1/8 tsp.
- Nutmeg – 1/8 tsp.
- Almond milk – ½ cup
- Stevia - 2 Tbsp.

Directions:

1. Scald the milk, then let it cool a little.

2. Break the egg into a bowl and beat it with the nutmeg.

3. Add the scalded milk, the vanilla, and the sweetener to taste. Mix well.

4. Place the bowl in a baking pan filled with ½ deep of water.

5. Bake for 30 minutes at 325F.

6. Serve.

Nutrition:

Calories: 167.3;

Fat: 9g;

Carb: 11g;

Phosphorus: 205mg;

Potassium: 249mg;

Sodium: 124mg;

Protein: 10g;

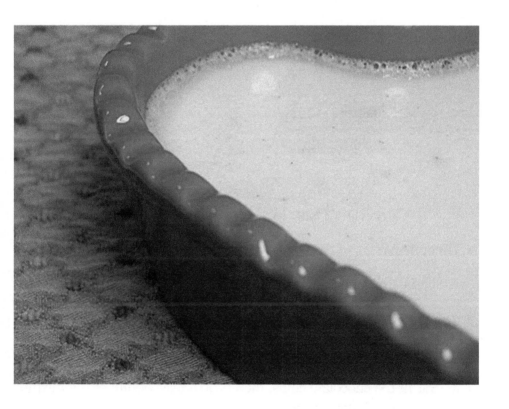

Chocolate Chip Cookies

Preparation Time: 7 minutes

Cooking Time: 10 minutes

Servings: 10

Ingredients:

- Semi-sweet chocolate chips – ½ cup

- Baking soda – ½ tsp.

- Vanilla – ½ tsp.

- Egg – 1

- Flour – 1 cup

- Margarine – ½ cup

- Stevia – 4 tsp.

Directions:

1. Sift the dry ingredients.

2. Cream the margarine, stevia, vanilla, and egg with a whisk.

3. Add flour mixture and beat well.

4. Stir in the chocolate chips, then drop a teaspoonful of the mixture over a greased baking sheet.

5. Bake the cookies for about 10 minutes at 375F.

6. Cool and serve.

Nutrition:

Calories: 106.2;

Fat: 7g;

Carb: 8.9g;

Phosphorus: 19mg;

Potassium: 28mg;

Sodium: 98mg;

Protein: 1.5g;

Baked Peaches with Cream Cheese

Preparation Time: 10 minutes

Cooking Time: 15 minutes

Servings: 4

Ingredients:

- Plain cream cheese – 1 cup

- Crushed meringue cookies – ½ cup

- Ground cinnamon – ¼ tsp.

- Pinch ground nutmeg

- Canned peach halves – 8, in juice

- Honey – 2 Tbsp.

Directions:

1. Preheat the oven to 350F.

2. Line a baking sheet with parchment paper. Set aside.

3. In a small bowl, stir together the meringue cookies, cream cheese, cinnamon, and nutmeg.

4. Spoon the cream cheese mixture evenly into the cavities in the peach halves.

5. Place the peaches on the baking sheet and bake for 15 minutes or

until the fruit is soft and the cheese is melted.

6. Remove the peaches from the baking sheet onto plates.

7. Drizzle with honey and serve.

Nutrition:

Calories: 260;

Fat: 20;

Carb: 19g;

Phosphorus: 74mg;

Potassium: 198mg;

Sodium: 216mg;

Protein: 4g;

Bread Pudding

Preparation Time: 15 minutes

Cooking Time: 40 minutes

Servings: 6

Ingredients:

- Unsalted butter, for greasing the baking dish
- Plain rice milk – 1 ½ cups
- Eggs – 2
- Egg whites – 2
- Honey – ¼ cup
- Pure vanilla extract – 1 tsp.
- Cubed white bread – 6 cups

Directions:

1. Grease an 8-by-8-inch baking dish with butter. Set it aside.

2. In a bowl, whisk together the eggs, egg whites, rice milk, honey, and vanilla.

3. Add the bread cubes and stir until the bread is coated.

4. Transfer the mixture to the baking dish and cover with plastic wrap.

5. Store the dish in the refrigerator for at least 3 hours.

6. Preheat the oven to 325F.

7. Take away the plastic wrap from the baking dish, bake the pudding for 35 to 40 minutes, or golden brown.

8. Serve.

Nutrition:

Calories: 167;

Fat: 3g;

Carb: 30g;

Phosphorus: 95mg;

Potassium: 93mg;

Sodium: 189mg;

Protein: 6g;

Strawberry Ice Cream

Preparation Time: 5 minutes

Cooking Time: 5 minutes

Servings: 3

Ingredients:

- Stevia – ½ cup

- Lemon juice – 1 Tbsp.

- Non-dairy coffee creamer – ¾ cup

- Strawberries – 10 oz.

- Crushed ice – 1 cup

Directions:

1. Blend everything in a blender until smooth.

2. Freeze until frozen.

3. Serve.

Nutrition:

Calories: 94.4;

Fat: 6g;

Carb: 8.3g;

Phosphorus: 25mg;

Potassium: 108mg;

Sodium: 25mg;

Protein: 1.3g;

Cinnamon Custard

Preparation Time: 20 minutes

Cooking Time: 1 hour

Servings: 6

Ingredients:

- Unsalted butter, for greasing the ramekins
- Plain rice milk – 1 ½ cups
- Eggs – 4
- Granulated sugar – ¼ cup
- Pure vanilla extract – 1 tsp.
- Ground cinnamon – ½ tsp.
- Cinnamon sticks for garnish

Directions:

1. Preheat the oven to 325F.

2. Lightly grease six ramekins and place them in a baking dish. Set aside.

3. In a large bowl, whisk together the eggs, rice milk, sugar, vanilla, and cinnamon until the mixture is smooth.

4. Pour the mixture through a fine sieve into a pitcher.

5. Evenly divide the custard mixture among the ramekins.

6. Fill the baking dish with hot water until the water reaches halfway up the sides of the ramekins.

7. Bake for 1 hour or until the custards are set, and a knife inserted in the center comes out clean.

8. Remove the custards from the oven and take the ramekins out of the water.

9. Cool on the wire racks for 1 hour, then chill for 1 hour.

10. Garnish with cinnamon sticks and serve.

Nutrition:

Calories: 110;

Fat: 4g;

Carb: 14g;

Phosphorus: 100mg;

Potassium: 64mg;

Sodium: 71mg;

Protein: 4g;

Cheesy Sausage Dip

Preparation Time: 10 Minutes

Cooking Time: 120 Minutes

Servings: 12

Ingredients:

- ½ pound ground Italian sausage
- ½ cup diced tomatoes
- Two green onions, sliced thin
- 4 ounces cream cheese, cubed
- 4 ounces pepper jack cheese, cubed
- 1 cup sour cream

Directions:

1. Brown the sausage in a skillet, wait for it to cook completely, then stir in the tomatoes.

2. Cook for 2 minutes, stirring often, thereafter, add in the green onions.

3. Line the bottom of a slow cooker with the cheeses, then spoon the sausage mixture on top.

4. Spoon the sour cream over the sausage, then cover and cook on high heat for 2 hours, stirring once halfway through.

5. Serve with celery sticks or pork rinds for dipping.

Nutrition:

Calories: 170

Fat: 15g

Protein: 7g

Net Carbs: 2g

Salted Kale Chips

Preparation Time: 10 Minutes

Cooking Time: 12 Minutes

Servings: 2

Ingredients:

- ½ bunch fresh kale
- 1 tablespoon olive oil
- Salt and pepper to taste

Directions:

1. Preheat the oven to 350o F and line a baking sheet with foil.

2. Pick the thick stems from the kale and then tear the leaves into pieces.

3. Toss the kale with olive oil and spread it on the baking sheet.

4. Bake for 10 to 12 minutes until crisp, then sprinkle with salt and pepper.

Nutrition:

Calories: 75
Fat: 7g
Protein: 1g
Net Carbs: 3g

Bacon Jalapeno Quick Bread

Preparation Time: 20 Minutes

Cooking Time: 45 Minutes

Servings: 10

Ingredients:

- Four slices of thick-cut bacon

- Three jalapeno peppers

- ½ cup coconut flour sifted

- ½ teaspoon baking soda

- ½ teaspoon salt

- Six large eggs, beaten

- ½ cup coconut oil, melted

- ¼ cup of water

Directions:

1. Preheat the oven to 400 F

2. Grease a loaf pan with cooking spray.

3. Spread the bacon and jalapenos on a baking sheet and roast for 10 minutes, stirring halfway through.

4. Crumble the bacon and cut the jalapenos in half to remove the seeds.

5. Combine the bacon and jalapeno in a food processor and pulse until well chopped.

6. Beat together the coconut flour, baking soda, and salt in a bowl.

7. Add the eggs, coconut oil, and water, then stir in the bacon and jalapenos.

8. Spread in the loaf pan, then bake for 40 to 45 minutes, until a knife inserted in the center comes out clean.

Nutrition:

Calories: 225

Fat: 19g

Protein: 8g

Net Carbs: 3g

Toasted Pumpkin Seeds

Preparation Time: 5 Minutes

Cooking Time: 5 Minutes

Servings: 2

Ingredients:

- ½ cup hulled pumpkin seeds

- 2 teaspoons coconut oil

- 2 teaspoons chili powder

- ½ teaspoon salt

Directions:

1. Heat a cast-iron skillet over medium heat.

2. Add the pumpkin seeds and let them cook until toasted, about 3 to 5 minutes, stirring often.

3. Remove from heat and stir in the coconut oil, chili powder, and salt.

4. Let the seeds cool, then store in an airtight container.

Nutrition:

Calories: 100
Fat: 8.5g
Protein: 5.5g
Net Carbs: 0.5g

Bacon-Wrapped Burger Bites

Preparation Time: 5 Minutes

Cooking Time: 60 Minutes

Servings: 6

Ingredients:

- 6 ounces ground beef (80% lean)
- ¼ teaspoon onion powder
- ¼ teaspoon garlic powder
- ¼ teaspoon ground cumin
- Salt and pepper to taste
- Six slices bacon, uncooked

Directions:

1. Preheat the oven to 350º F
2. Combine the onion powder, garlic powder, cumin, salt, and pepper in a bowl.
3. Add the beef and stir until well combined.
4. Divide the ground beef mixture into six even portions and roll them into balls.
5. Wrap each ball with a slice of bacon and place it on the baking sheet.

6. Bake for 60 minutes until the bacon is crisp and the beef is cooked through.

Nutrition:

Calories: 150

Fat: 10g

Protein: 16g

Net Carbs: 0.5g

Almond Sesame Crackers

Preparation Time: 10 Minutes

Cooking Time: 15 Minutes

Servings: 6

Ingredients:

- 1 ½ cups almond flour
- ½ cup sesame seeds
- 1 teaspoon dried oregano
- ½ teaspoon salt
- 1 large egg, whisked
- 1 tablespoon coconut oil, melted

Directions:

1. Preheat the oven to 350o F
2. Whisk together the almond flour, sesame seeds, oregano, and salt in a bowl.
3. Add the eggs and coconut oil, stirring into a soft dough.
4. Sandwich the dough between two sheets of parchment and roll to 1/8" thickness.
5. Cut into squares and arrange them on the baking sheet.

6. Bake for 10 to 12 minutes or wait until browned around the edges.

Nutrition:

Calories: 145

Fat: 12.5g

Protein: 5g

Net Carbs: 2g

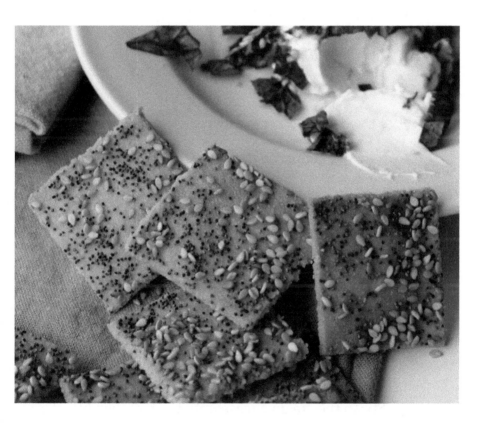

Cauliflower Cheese Dip

Preparation Time: 5 Minutes

Cooking Time: 15 Minutes

Servings: 6

Ingredients:

- One small head cauliflower, chopped

- ¾ cup chicken broth

- ¼ teaspoon ground cumin

- ¼ teaspoon chili powder

- ¼ teaspoon garlic powder

- Salt and pepper to taste

- 1/3 cup cream cheese, chopped

- Two tablespoons canned coconut milk

Directions:

1. Combine the cauliflower and chicken broth in a saucepan and simmer until the cauliflower is tender.

2. Add the cumin, chili powder, and garlic powder, then season with salt and pepper.

3. Stir in the cream cheese until melted, then blend everything with an immersion blender.

4. Whisk in the coconut milk, then spoon into a serving bowl.

5. Serve with sliced celery sticks.

Nutrition:

Calories: 75

Fat: 6g

Protein: 2.5g

Net Carbs: 2g

Raspberry Muffins

Preparation Time: 10 Minutes

Cooking Time: 25 Minutes

Servings: 12

Ingredients:

- ½ cup and 2 tablespoons whole-wheat flour
- 1 ½ cup raspberries, fresh and more for decorating
- 1 cup white whole-wheat flour
- 1/8 teaspoon salt
- ¾ cup of coconut sugar
- 2 teaspoons baking powder
- 1 teaspoon apple cider vinegar
- 1 ¼ cups water
- ½ cup olive oil

Directions:

1. Switch on the oven, then set it to 400 degrees F and let it preheat.

2. Meanwhile, take a large bowl, place both flours in it, add salt and baking powder and then stir until combined.

3. Take a medium bowl, add oil to it, and then whisk in the sugar until dissolved.

4. Whisk in vinegar and water until blended, slowly stir in flour mixture until smooth batter comes together, and then fold in berries.

5. Take a 12-cups muffin pan, grease it with oil, fill evenly with the prepared mixture and then put a raspberry on top of each muffin.

6. Bake the muffins for 25 minutes until the top golden brown, and then serve.

Nutrition:

Calories: 109 Cal;

Fat: 3.4 g;

Protein: 2.1 g;

Carbs: 17.6 g;

Fiber: 1 g

Chocolate Chip Cake

Preparation Time: 10 Minutes

Cooking Time: 50 Minutes

Servings: 10

Ingredients:

- 2 cups white whole-wheat flour
- ¼ teaspoon baking soda
- 1/3 cup coconut sugar
- 2 teaspoons baking powder
- ½ teaspoon salt
- ½ cup chocolate chips, vegan
- 1 teaspoon vanilla extract, unsweetened
- 1 tablespoon applesauce
- 1 teaspoon apple cider vinegar
- ¼ cup melted coconut oil
- ½ teaspoon almond extract, unsweetened
- 1 cup almond milk, unsweetened

Directions:

1. Switch on the oven, then set it to 360 degrees F and let it preheat.

2. Meanwhile, take a 9-by-5 inches loaf pan, grease it with oil, and then set aside until required.

3. Take a large bowl, add sugar to it, pour in oil, vanilla and almond extract, vinegar, apple sauce, and milk, and then whisk until well combined.

4. Take a large bowl, place flour in it, add salt, baking powder, and soda, and then stir until mixed.

5. Stir the flour mixture into the milk mixture until smooth batter comes together, and then fold in 1/3 cup of chocolate chips.

6. Spoon the batter into the loaf pan, scatter remaining chocolate chips on top and then bake for 50 minutes.

7. When done, let the bread cool for 10 minutes and then cut it into slices.

8. Serve straight away.

Nutrition:

Calories: 218 Cal;

Fat: 8 g;

Protein: 3.4 g;

Carbs: 32 g;

Fiber: 2 g

Coffee Cake

Preparation Time: 10 Minutes

Cooking Time: 45 Minutes

Servings: 9

Ingredients:

For the Cake:

- 1/3 cup coconut sugar
- 1 teaspoon vanilla extract, unsweetened
- ¼ cup olive oil
- 1/8 teaspoon almond extract, unsweetened
- 1 ¾ cup white whole-wheat flour
- 2 teaspoons baking powder
- ½ teaspoon salt
- ¼ teaspoon baking soda
- 1 teaspoon apple cider vinegar
- 1 tablespoon applesauce
- 1 cup almond milk, unsweetened

For the Streusel:

- ½ cup white whole-wheat flour

- 2 teaspoons cinnamon

- 1/3 cup coconut sugar

- ½ teaspoon salt

- 2 tablespoons olive oil

- 1 tablespoon coconut butter

Directions:

1. Switch on the oven, then set it to 350 degrees F and let it preheat.

2. Meanwhile, take a large bowl, pour in milk, add applesauce, vinegar, sugar, oil, vanilla, and almond extract and then whisk until blended.

3. Take a medium bowl, place flour in it, add salt, baking powder, and soda and then stir until mixed.

4. Stir the flour mixture into the milk mixture until smooth batter comes together, and then spoon the mixture into a loaf pan lined with parchment paper.

5. Prepare streusel and for this, take a medium bowl, place flour in it, and then add sugar, salt, and cinnamon.

6. Stir until mixed, and then mix butter and oil with fingers until the crumble mixture comes together.

7. Spread the prepared streusel on top of the batter of the cake and then bake for 45 minutes until the top turn golden brown and cake have thoroughly cooked.

8. When done, let the cake rest in its pan for 10 minutes, remove it to cool completely and then cut it into slices.

9. Serve straight away.

Nutrition:

Calories: 259 Cal;

Fat: 10 g;

Protein: 3 g;

Carbs: 37 g;

Fiber: 1 g

Chocolate Marble Cake

Preparation Time: 15 Minutes

Cooking Time: 50 Minutes

Servings: 8

Ingredients:

- 1 ½ cup white whole-wheat flour

- 1 tablespoon flaxseed meal

- 2 ½ tablespoons cocoa powder

- ¼ teaspoon salt

- 4 tablespoons chopped walnuts

- 1 teaspoon baking powder

- 2/3 cup coconut sugar

- ¼ teaspoon baking soda

- 1 teaspoon vanilla extract, unsweetened

- 3 tablespoons peanut butter

- ¼ cup olive oil

- 1 cup almond milk, unsweetened

Directions:

1. Switch on the oven, then set it to 350 degrees F and let it preheat.

2. Meanwhile, take a medium bowl, place flour in it, add salt, baking powder, and soda in it and then stir until mixed.

3. Take a large bowl, pour in milk, add sugar, flaxseed, oil, and vanilla, whisk until sugar has dissolved, and then whisk in flour mixture until smooth batter comes together.

4. Spoon half of the prepared batter in a medium bowl, add cocoa powder and then stir until combined.

5. Add peanut butter into the other bowl and then stir until combined.

6. Take a loaf pan, line it with a parchment sheet, spoon half of the chocolate batter in it, and then spread it evenly.

7. Layer the chocolate batter with half of the peanut butter batter, cover with the remaining chocolate batter and then layer with the remaining peanut butter batter.

8. Make swirls into the batter with a toothpick, smooth the top with a spatula, sprinkle walnuts on top, and then bake for 50 minutes until done.

9. When done, let the cake rest in its pan for 10 minutes, then remove it to cool completely and cut it into slices.

10. Serve straight away.

Nutrition:

Calories: 299 Cal;

Fat: 14 g;

Protein: 6 g;

Carbs: 39 g;

Fiber: 3 g

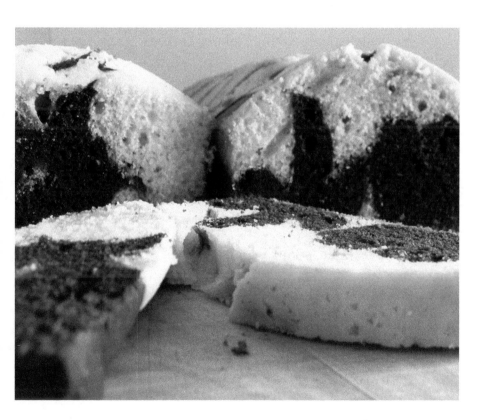

Chocolate Chip Cookies

Preparation Time: 10 Minutes

Cooking Time: 10 Minutes

Servings: 11

Ingredients:

- 1 ¼ cups white whole-wheat flour
- 1 ½ tablespoon flax seeds
- ½ teaspoon baking soda
- ½ cup of coconut sugar
- ¼ teaspoon of sea salt
- ¼ cup powdered coconut sugar
- 1 teaspoon baking powder
- 2 teaspoons vanilla extract, unsweetened
- 4 ½ tablespoons water
- ½ cup of coconut oil
- 1 cup chocolate chips, vegan

Directions:

1. Take a large bowl, place flax seeds in it, stir in water and then let the mixture rest for 5 minutes until creamy.

2. Then add remaining ingredients into the flax seed's mixture except for flour and chocolate chips and then beat until light batter comes together.

3. Beat in flour, ¼ cup at a time, until smooth batter comes together, and then fold in chocolate chips.

4. Use an ice cream scoop to scoop the batter onto a baking sheet lined with parchment sheet with some distance between cookies and then bake for 10 minutes until cookies turn golden brown.

5. When done, let the cookies cool on the baking sheet for 3 minutes and then cool completely on the wire rack for 5 minutes.

6. Serve straight away.

Nutrition:

Calories: 141 Cal;

Fat: 7 g;

Protein: 1 g;

Carbs: 17 g;

Fiber: 2 g

Lemon Cake

Preparation Time: 10 Minutes

Cooking Time: 50 Minutes

Servings: 9

Ingredients:

- 1 ½ cup white whole-wheat flour
- 1 ½ teaspoon baking powder
- 2 tablespoons almond flour
- 1 lemon, zested
- ¼ teaspoon baking soda
- 1/8 teaspoon turmeric powder
- 1/3 teaspoon salt
- ¼ teaspoon vanilla extract, unsweetened
- 1/3 cup lemon juice
- ½ cup maple syrup
- ¼ cup olive oil
- ¼ cup of water

For the Frosting:

- 1 tablespoon lemon juice

- 1/8 teaspoon salt

- ¼ cup maple syrup

- 2 tablespoons powdered sugar

- 6 ounces vegan cream cheese, softened

Directions:

1. Switch on the oven, then set it to 350 degrees F and let it preheat.

2. Take a large bowl, pour in water, lemon juice, and oil, add vanilla extract and maple syrup, and whisk until blended.

3. Whisk in flour, ¼ cup at a time, until smooth, and then whisk in almond flour, salt, turmeric, lemon zest, baking soda, and powder until well combined.

4. Take a loaf pan, grease it with oil, spoon prepared batter in it, and then bake for 50 minutes.

5. Meanwhile, prepare the frosting and for this, take a small bowl, place all of its ingredients in it, whisk until smooth, and then let it chill until required.

6. When the cake has cooked, let it cool for 10 minutes in its pan and then let it cool completely on the wire rack.

7. Spread the prepared frosting on top of the cake, slice the cake, and then serve.

Nutrition:

Calories: 275 Cal;

Fat: 12 g;

Protein: 3 g;

Carbs: 38 g;

Fiber: 1 g

Banana Muffins

Preparation Time: 10 Minutes

Cooking Time: 30 Minutes

Servings: 12

Ingredients:

- 1 ½ cups mashed banana
- 1 ½ cups and 2 tablespoons white whole-wheat flour, divided
- ¼ cup of coconut sugar
- ¾ cup rolled oats, divided
- 1 teaspoon ginger powder
- 1 tablespoon ground cinnamon, divided
- 2 teaspoons baking powder
- ½ teaspoon salt
- 1 teaspoon baking soda
- 1 tablespoon vanilla extract, unsweetened
- ½ cup maple syrup
- 1 tablespoon rum
- ½ cup of coconut oil

Directions:

1. Switch on the oven, then set it to 350 degrees F and let it preheat.

2. Meanwhile, take a medium bowl, place 1 ½ cup flour in it, add ½ cup oars, ginger, baking powder and soda, salt, and 2 teaspoons cinnamon and then stir until mixed.

3. Place ¼ cup of coconut oil in a heatproof bowl, melt it in the microwave oven and then whisk in maple syrup until combined.

4. Add mashed banana along with rum and vanilla, stir until combined, and then whisk this mixture into the flour mixture until smooth batter comes together.

5. Take a separate medium bowl, place remaining oats and flour in it, add cinnamon, coconut sugar, and coconut oil and then stir with a fork until crumbly mixture comes together.

6. Take a 12-cups muffin pan, fill evenly with prepared batter, top with oats mixture, and then bake for 30 minutes until firm and the top turn golden brown.

7. When done, let the muffins cool for 5 minutes in its pan and then cool the muffins completely before serving.

Nutrition:

Calories: 240 Cal;

Fat: 9.3 g;

Protein: 2.6 g;

Carbs: 35.4 g;

Fiber: 2 g

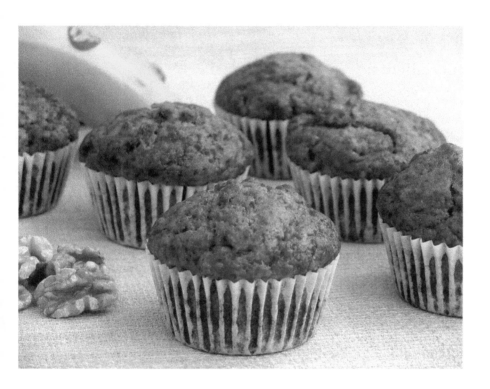

No-Bake Cookies

Preparation Time: 30 Minutes

Cooking Time: 0 Minutes

Servings: 9

Ingredients:

- 1 cup rolled oats

- ¼ cup of cocoa powder

- 1/8 teaspoon salt

- 1 teaspoon vanilla extract, unsweetened

- ¼ cup and 2 tablespoons peanut butter, divided

- 6 tablespoons coconut oil, divided

- ¼ cup and 1 tablespoon maple syrup, divided

Directions:

1. Take a small saucepan, place it over low heat, add 5 tablespoons of coconut oil and then let it melt.

2. Whisk in 2 tablespoons peanut butter, salt, 1 teaspoon vanilla extract, and ¼ cup each of cocoa powder and maple syrup, and then whisk until well combined.

3. Remove pan from heat, stir in oats and then spoon the mixture evenly into 9 cups of a muffin pan.

4. Wipe clean the pan, return it over low heat, add remaining coconut oil, maple syrup, and peanut butter, stir until combined, and then cook for 2 minutes until thoroughly warmed.

5. Drizzle the peanut butter sauce over the oat mixture in the muffin pan and then let it freeze for 20 minutes or more until set.

6. Serve straight away.

Nutrition:

Calories: 213 Cal;

Fat: 14.8 g;

Protein: 4 g;

Carbs: 17.3 g;

Fiber: 2.1 g

Peanut Butter and Oat Bars

Preparation Time: 40 Minutes

Cooking Time: 8 Minutes

Servings: 8

Ingredients:

- 1 cup rolled oats

- 1/8 teaspoon salt

- ¼ cup chocolate chips, vegan

- ¼ cup maple syrup

- 1 cup peanut butter

Directions:

1. Take a medium saucepan, place it over medium heat, add peanut butter, salt, and maple syrup and then whisk until combined and thickened; this will take 5 minutes.

2. Remove pan from heat, place oats in a bowl, pour peanut butter mixture on it and then stir until well combined.

3. Take an 8-by-6 inches baking dish, line it with a parchment sheet, spoon the oats mixture in it, and then spread evenly, pressing the mixture into the dish.

4. Sprinkle the chocolate chips on top, press them into the bar mixture and then let the mixture rest in the refrigerator for 30 minutes or more until set.

5. When ready to eat, cut the bar mixture into even size pieces and then serve.

Nutrition:

Calories: 274 Cal;

Fat: 17 g;

Protein: 10 g;

Carbs: 19 g;

Fiber: 3 g

Baked Apples

Preparation Time: 5 Minutes

Cooking Time: 20 Minutes

Servings: 4

Ingredients:

- 6 medium apples, peeled, cut into chunks

- 1 teaspoon ground cinnamon

- 2 tablespoons melted coconut oil

Directions:

1. Switch on the oven, then set it to 350 degrees F and let it preheat.

2. Take a medium baking dish, and then spread apple pieces in it.

3. Take a small bowl, place coconut oil in it, stir in cinnamon, drizzle this mixture over apples and then toss until coated.

4. Place the baking dish into the oven and then bake for 20 minutes or more until apples turn soft, stirring halfway.

5. Serve straight away.

Nutrition:

Calories: 170 Cal;

Fat: 3.8 g;

Protein: 0.5 g;

Carbs: 31 g;

Fiber: 5.5 g

Chocolate Strawberry Shake

Preparation Time: 5 Minutes

Cooking Time: 0 Minutes

Servings: 2

Ingredients:

- 2 cups almond milk, unsweetened

- 4 bananas, peeled, frozen

- 4 tablespoons cocoa powder

- 2 cups strawberries, frozen

Directions:

1. Place all the ingredients into the jar of a high-speed food processor or blender in the order stated in the ingredients list and then cover it with the lid.

2. Pulse for 1 minute until smooth, and then serve.

Nutrition:

Calories: 208 Cal;

Fat: 0.2 g;

Protein: 12.4 g;

Carbs: 26.2 g;

Fiber: 1.4 g

Chocolate Clusters

Preparation Time: 15 Minutes

Cooking Time: 0 Minutes

Servings: 12

Ingredients:

- 1 cup chopped dark chocolate, vegan

- 1 cup cashews, roasted, salt

- 1 teaspoon sea salt flakes

Directions:

1. Take a large baking sheet, line it with wax paper, and then set aside until required.

2. Take a medium bowl, place chocolate in it, and then microwave for 1 minute.

3. Stir the chocolate and then continue microwaving it at 1-minute intervals until chocolate melts completely, stirring at every interval.

4. When melted, stir the chocolate to bring it to 90 degrees F and then stir in cashews.

5. Scoop the walnut-chocolate mixture on the prepared baking sheet, ½ tablespoons per cluster, and then sprinkle with salt.

6. Let the clusters stand at room temperature until harden and then serve.

Nutrition:

Calories: 79.4 Cal;

Fat: 6.6 g;

Protein: 1 g;

Carbs: 5.8 g;

Fiber: 1.1 g

Banana Coconut Cookies

Preparation Time: 40 Minutes

Cooking Time: 0 Minutes

Servings: 8

Ingredients:

- 1 ½ cup shredded coconut, unsweetened

- 1 cup mashed banana

Directions:

1. Switch on the oven, then set it to 350 degrees F and let it preheat.

2. Take a medium bowl, place the mashed banana in it and then stir in coconut until well combined.

3. Take a large baking sheet, line it with a parchment sheet, and then scoop the prepared mixture on it, 2 tablespoons of mixture per cookie.

4. Place the baking sheet into the refrigerator and then let it cool for 30 minutes or more until harden.

5. Serve straight away.

Nutrition:

Calories: 51 Cal;

Fat: 3 g;

Protein: 0.2 g;

Carbs: 4 g;

Fiber: 1 g

Chocolate Pots

Preparation Time: 4 Hours 10 Minutes

Cooking Time: 3 Minutes

Servings: 4

Ingredients:

- 6 ounces chocolate, unsweetened

- 1 cup Medjool dates, pitted

- 1 ¾ cups almond milk, unsweetened

Directions:

1. Cut the chocolate into small pieces, place them in a heatproof bowl and then microwave for 2 to 3 minutes until melt completely, stirring every minute.

2. Place dates in a blender, pour in the milk, and then pulse until smooth.

3. Add chocolate into the blender and then pulse until combined.

4. Divide the mixture into the small mason jars and then let them rest for 4 hours until set.

5. Serve straight away.

Nutrition:

Calories: 321 Cal;

Fat: 19 g;

Protein: 6 g;

Carbs: 34 g;

Fiber: 4 g

Maple and Tahini Fudge

Preparation Time: 2 Hours

Cooking Time: 3 Minutes

Servings: 15

Ingredients:

- 1 cup dark chocolate chips, vegan

- ¼ cup maple syrup

- ½ cup tahini

Directions:

1. Take a heatproof bowl, place chocolate chips in it and then microwave for 2 to 3 minutes until melt completely, stirring every minute.

2. When melted, remove the chocolate bowl from the oven and then whisk in maple syrup and tahini until smooth.

3. Take a 4-by-8 inches baking dish, line it with wax paper, spoon the chocolate mixture in it and then press it into the baking dish.

4. Cover with another sheet with wax paper, press it down until smooth, and then let the fudge rest for 1 hour in the freezer until set.

5. Then cut the fudge into 15 squares and serve.

Nutrition:

Calories: 110.7 Cal;

Fat: 5.3 g;

Protein: 2.2 g;

Carbs: 15.1 g;

Fiber: 1.6 g

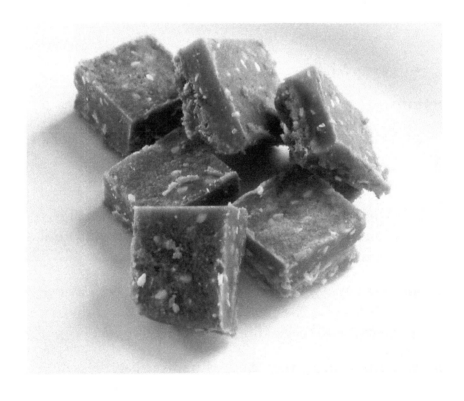

Creaseless

Preparation Time: 5 Minutes

Cooking Time: 0 Minutes

Servings: 5

Ingredients:

- 3 tablespoons agave syrup

- 1 cup coconut milk, unsweetened

- ½ teaspoon vanilla extract, unsweetened

- 1 cup of orange juice

Directions:

1. Place all the ingredients in a food processor or blender and then pulse until combined.

2. Pour the mixture into five molds of Popsicle pan, insert a stick into each mold and then let it freeze for a minimum of 4 hours until hard.

3. Serve when ready.

Nutrition:

Calories: 152 Cal;
Fat: 10 g;
Protein: 1 g;
Carbs: 16 g;
Fiber: 1 g

Peanut Butter, Nut, and Fruit Cookies

Preparation Time: 30 Minutes

Cooking Time: 0 Minutes

Servings: 25

Ingredients:

- ¾ cup rolled oats

- ¼ cup chopped peanuts

- ½ cup coconut flakes, unsweetened

- ¼ cup and 2 tablespoons chopped cranberries, dried

- ¼ cup sliced almonds

- ¼ cup and 2 tablespoons raisins

- ¼ cup maple syrup

- ¾ cup peanut butter

Directions:

1. Take a baking sheet, line it with wax paper, and then set it aside until required.

2. Take a large bowl, place oats, almonds, and coconut flakes in it, add ¼ cup each of cranberries and raisins, and then stir until combined.

3. Add maple syrup and peanut butter, stir until well combined, and then scoop the mixture on the prepared baking sheet with some distance between them.

4. Flatten each scoop of cookie mixture slightly, press remaining cranberries and raisins into each cookie, and then let it chill for 20 minutes until firm.

5. Serve straight away.

Nutrition:

Calories: 140 Cal;

Fat: 7 g;

Protein: 3 g;

Carbs: 18 g;

Fiber: 5 g

Chocolate Covered Dates

Preparation Time: 10 Minutes

Cooking Time: 3 Minutes

Servings: 8

Ingredients:

- 16 Medjool dates, pitted
- ½ teaspoon of sea salt
- ¾ cup almonds
- 1 teaspoon coconut oil
- 8 ounces chocolate chips, vegan

Directions:

1. Take a medium baking sheet, line it with parchment paper, and then set aside until required.

2. Place an almond into the pit of each date and then wrap the date tightly around it.

3. Place chocolate chips in a heatproof bowl, add oil, and then microwave for 2 to 3 minutes until chocolate melts, stirring every minute.

4. Working on one date at a time, dip each date into the chocolate mixture and then place it onto the prepared baking sheet.

5. Sprinkle salt over the prepared dates and then let them rest in the refrigerator for 1 hour until chocolate is firm.

6. Serve straight away.

Nutrition:

Calories: 179 Cal;

Fat: 7.7 g;

Protein: 3 g;

Carbs: 28.5 g;

Fiber: 3 g

Hot Chocolate

Preparation Time: 5 Minutes

Cooking Time: 10 Minutes

Servings: 4

Ingredients:

- ¼ cup of cocoa powder

- 1/8 teaspoon salt

- ½ teaspoon vanilla extract, unsweetened

- ¼ cup of coconut sugar

- 3 cups almond milk, unsweetened

Directions:

1. Take a medium saucepan, add salt, sugar, and cocoa powder in it, whisk until combined, and then whisk in milk.

2. Place the pan over medium-high heat and then bring the milk mixture to a simmer and turn hot, continue whisking.

3. Divide the hot chocolate evenly into four mugs and then serve.

Nutrition:

Calories: 137 Cal;

Fat: 3 g;

Protein: 6 g;

Carbs: 21 g;

Fiber: 2 g

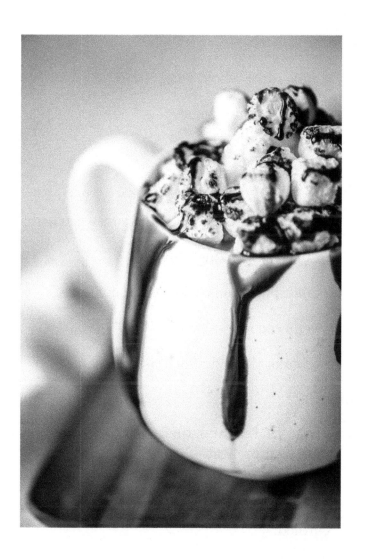

Vanilla Cupcakes

Preparation Time: 10 Minutes

Cooking Time: 20 Minutes

Servings: 18

Ingredients:

- 2 cups white whole-wheat flour

- 1 cup of coconut sugar

- ½ teaspoon salt

- 2 teaspoons baking powder

- 1 ¼ teaspoons vanilla extract, unsweetened

- ½ teaspoon baking soda

- 1 tablespoon apple cider vinegar

- ½ cup coconut oil, melted

- 1 ½ cups almond milk, unsweetened

Directions:

1. Switch on the oven, then set it to 350 degrees F, and then let it preheat.

2. Meanwhile, take a medium bowl, place vinegar in it, stir in milk, and then let it stand for 5 minutes until curdled.

3. Take a large bowl, place flour in it, add salt, baking soda and powder, and sugar and then stir until mixed.

4. Take a separate large bowl, pour in curdled milk mixture, add vanilla and coconut oil and then whisk until combined.

5. Whisk almond milk mixture into the flour mixture until smooth batter comes together, and then spoon the mixture into two 12-cups muffin pans lined with muffin cups.

6. Bake the muffins for 15 to 20 minutes until firm and the top turn golden brown, and then let them cool on the wire rack completely.

7. Serve straight away.

Nutrition:

Calories: 152.4 Cal;

Fat: 6.4 g;

Protein: 1.5 g;

Carbs: 22.6 g;

Fiber: 0.5 g

Stuffed Dried Figs

Preparation Time: 20 Minutes

Cooking Time: 0 Minutes

Servings: 4

Ingredients:

- 12 dried figs

- 2 Tbsps. thyme honey

- 2 Tbsps. sesame seeds

- 24 walnut halves

Directions:

1. Cut off the tough stalk ends of the figs.

2. Slice open each fig.

3. Stuff the fig openings with two walnut halves and close

4. Arrange the figs on a plate, drizzle with honey, and sprinkle the sesame seeds on it.

5. Serve.

Nutrition:

Calories: 110kcal
Carbs: 26
Fat: 3g,
Protein: 1g